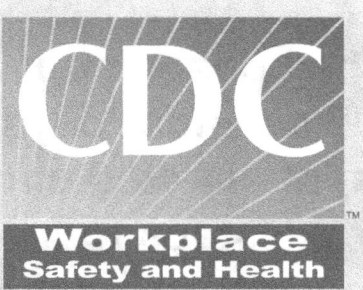

Knowledge, Attitudes, and Practices Regarding Influenza Vaccination Among Employees at Child Care Centers — Ohio

Marie A. de Perio, MD
Douglas M. Wiegand, PhD
Stefanie M. Evans, MA

Health Hazard Evaluation Report
HETA 2010-0025-3121
February 2011

DEPARTMENT OF HEALTH AND HUMAN SERVICES
Centers for Disease Control and Prevention

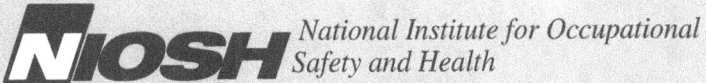

National Institute for Occupational
Safety and Health

The employer shall post a copy of this report for a period of 30 calendar days at or near the workplace(s) of affected employees. The employer shall take steps to insure that the posted determinations are not altered, defaced, or covered by other material during such period. [37 FR 23640, November 7, 1972, as amended at 45 FR 2653, January 14, 1980].

CONTENTS

ABBREVIATIONS

ACIP	Advisory Committee on Immunization Practices
CDC	Centers for Disease Control and Prevention
FDA	Food and Drug Administration
GEE	Generalized estimating equations
NAICS	North American Industry Classification System
NAEYC	National Association for the Education of Young Children
NIOSH	National Institute for Occupational Safety and Health
pH1N1	2009 pandemic influenza A (H1N1)
VAERS	Vaccine Adverse Event Reporting System
VSD	Vaccine Safety Datalink

In November 2009, the National Institute for Occupational Safety and Health (NIOSH) received a technical assistance request from the Department of Jobs and Family Services at an Ohio county. The request asked for NIOSH assistance in examining rates of 2009 pandemic influenza A (H1N1) (pH1N1) and seasonal influenza (also known as the flu) vaccination among employees at licensed child care centers in the county. The request also asked for assistance in assessing knowledge of and attitudes towards these two vaccines.

What NIOSH Did

- We surveyed 384 employees at 32 licensed child care centers.

- We asked employees what they knew and thought about the two vaccines. We also asked whether they had gotten or planned to get the vaccines.

What NIOSH Found

- We found low rates of pH1N1 (12%) and seasonal influenza (25%) vaccination among child care center employees.

- The most common reasons for not getting either vaccine were beliefs that employees did not need the vaccine, that the vaccine did not work, and that the vaccine was not safe.

- People who had positive opinions about the vaccine or felt pressure from others to get the vaccine were more likely to have been vaccinated.

What Employers and Directors Can Do

- Work with the county health department or local healthcare providers to offer the vaccine at no cost at child care centers.

- Educate employees about the flu. Focus on employees' risk of infection, the efficacy and safety of the vaccine, and their responsibility to get vaccinated.

- Consider requiring employees to get the flu vaccine as part of a comprehensive flu prevention program. If this is not feasible, encourage employees to get vaccinated.

What Employees Can Do

- Get the seasonal flu vaccine every year. Vaccination is the most effective way to avoid getting the flu, which can cause lost time from work, serious illness, and death.

- Stay informed. Get information about the flu and the flu vaccine from reliable sources.

This page intentionally left blank.

SUMMARY

NIOSH investigators examined the knowledge, attitudes, and receipt of seasonal influenza and pH1N1 influenza vaccines among child care center employees. We found low rates of pH1N1 and seasonal influenza vaccination. The most common reasons for not receiving either vaccine included believing that employees did not need the vaccine, that the vaccine did not work, and that the vaccine was not safe.

In November 2009, NIOSH received a technical assistance request from the Department of Jobs and Family Services at an Ohio county. The request asked for NIOSH assistance in examining rates of pH1N1 and seasonal influenza vaccination and in assessing knowledge of and attitudes towards these two vaccines among employees at licensed child care centers in the county.

We performed a cross-sectional survey among employees of 32 randomly selected licensed child care centers. From January 30–March 1, 2010, we surveyed employees about personal and work characteristics, pertinent medical history, receipt of or intention to receive the pH1N1 and seasonal influenza vaccines, and knowledge about and attitudes towards each vaccine.

Of 403 invited child care employees, 384 (95%) completed a survey. Forty-five (12%) respondents reported having received the pH1N1 vaccine. Eighty-five (22%) respondents reported having received the seasonal influenza vaccine. The most common reason for receiving either vaccine was to protect oneself or one's family.

For both vaccines, among unvaccinated respondents, 19% reported that they intended to get the vaccine, and 81% reported that they did not intend to do so. The most common reasons cited for not intending to receive either vaccine were "I don't think the vaccine will keep me from getting the flu" and "I don't think I need the vaccine."

Respondents who cared for toddlers or children 13 months–3 years, had some college or higher as the highest level of education, had positive attitudes towards the vaccine, felt external pressure from others to get the vaccine, and felt personal control over whether or not to get the vaccine were more likely to have received the pH1N1 vaccine than those who did not have these characteristics. Respondents who believed in the efficacy of the vaccine, had positive attitudes towards the vaccine, felt external pressure from others to get the vaccine, and felt personal control over whether or not to get the vaccine were more likely to have received the seasonal influenza vaccine than those who did not have these characteristics.

We found that employees at child care centers in the county had low rates of pH1N1 and seasonal influenza vaccination. Misconceptions about the need for the vaccines and the efficacy and safety of the vaccines were the most common reasons cited for not receiving either vaccine.

SUMMARY
(CONTINUED)

Vaccination remains the most effective method to prevent influenza, which can cause lost work time, serious illness, and death. Annual influenza vaccination of all persons aged ≥ 6 months is now recommended for the 2010–2011 influenza season. We recommend that efforts to improve vaccination rates among child care providers include notification of vaccination campaigns through media and public health messages addressing the most frequent antivaccination ideas. Educational interventions in the form of training that focuses on child care providers' risk for infection, the efficacy and safety profile of the vaccine, and providers' responsibility to get vaccinated should also be considered for this group. Employers should consider requiring influenza vaccination for their employees as part of a comprehensive influenza prevention program. If this is not feasible, then employers should encourage employees to get the vaccine.

Keywords: NAICS 624410 (Child Day Care Services), influenza, vaccination, child care, H1N1, pandemic, infection

INTRODUCTION

On November 9, 2009, NIOSH received a technical assistance request from the Department of Jobs and Family Services at an Ohio county. The request asked for NIOSH assistance in examining rates of pH1N1 and seasonal influenza vaccination and in assessing knowledge of and attitudes towards these two vaccines among employees at licensed child care centers in the county.

Background on Licensed Child Care Centers in the County

The county is located in southwestern Ohio and covers 407 square miles. It contains a major metropolitan area, and its population was estimated to be 855,062 in 2009 [U.S. Census Bureau 2010]. In 2009, 4,332 child care facilities, including centers and homes, were licensed in Ohio and served 279,674 children. Approximately 28,525 individuals are employed in these licensed facilities [ODJFS 2009]. The Bureau of Child Care and Development in the Ohio Department of Jobs and Family Services is responsible for inspecting, licensing, certifying, and regulating child care facilities in the state.

As of January 2010, the county had 362 licensed child care centers with thousands of employees. Of these 362 centers, 135 served infants younger than 18 months. The Department of Jobs and Family Services at the county administers federal, state, and local programs in the areas of child support, children's services, family and adult assistance, child care, adult protection, and workforce development. It contracts with more than 1,500 home providers and centers to cover part of the cost of child care for eligible low- and moderate-income families.

Child care centers in Ohio may participate in at least two voluntary quality control programs. NAEYC, an organization that focuses on the quality of education and developmental services for all children from birth through age 8, operates a national, voluntary accreditation program that has set professional standards for early childhood education programs since 1985. In the county, 22 licensed child care centers participated in this accreditation program. Step Up To Quality is another voluntary quality rating system for Ohio Department of Jobs and Family Services-licensed child care programs. It recognizes early care and education programs that exceed quality benchmarks over and above Ohio's licensing standards. In 2009, 880 early childhood programs in

Ohio participated in the Step Up to Quality program. In the county, 64 licensed child care centers participated in this program in 2009.

Background on Influenza

Influenza, commonly known as the flu, is a contagious respiratory illness caused by influenza viruses. Influenza viruses are thought to be spread mainly by droplets made when people with influenza cough, sneeze, or talk. Less often, a person might also get influenza by touching a surface or object that has influenza virus on it and then touching their own mouth, eyes, or nose [Wright and Webster 2001]. Evidence for airborne transmission (or aerosolization of small particles that may remain suspended in air for long periods) also exists [Bridges et al. 2003; Blachere et al. 2009; Lindsley et al. 2010a,b]. Influenza can cause mild to severe illness and can lead to death. Symptoms of influenza include fever, chills, cough, sore throat, runny or stuffy nose, muscle or body aches, headaches, fatigue, vomiting, and diarrhea [Nicholson 1992].

Complications of influenza include bacterial pneumonia, ear infections, sinus infections, dehydration, and worsening of chronic medical conditions [CDC 2010e]. Individuals at higher risk for developing influenza-related complications include children younger than 5 years (especially children younger than 2 years), adults 65 years of age and older, pregnant women, and people with chronic medical conditions (asthma; chronic lung disease; neurological conditions; heart disease; blood, endocrine, kidney, liver, and metabolic disorders; weakened immune system due to human immunodeficiency virus, cancer, or medication; and morbid obesity) [CDC 2010e]. In the United States, more than 200,000 people each year are hospitalized for influenza-related illnesses [Thompson et al. 2004]. CDC estimates that from 1976 to 2007, influenza-associated deaths ranged from a low of about 3,000 to a high of about 49,000 people per year in the United States [CDC 2010a].

The pH1N1 virus, also referred to as "swine flu," was first detected in humans in the United States in April 2009. On June 11, 2009, the World Health Organization signaled that a pandemic of pH1N1 was underway. The CDC estimated that, between April 2009 and April 2010, 43–89 million cases of pH1N1, 195,000–403,000 pH1N1-related hospitalizations, and 8,870–18,300 pH1N1-related deaths occurred [CDC 2010i].

Spread of the pH1N1 virus is thought to occur in the same way that seasonal influenza spreads [CDC 2009a]. The symptoms of pH1N1 infection include fever, cough, sore throat, runny or stuffy nose, body aches, headache, chills, and fatigue. Some patients have vomiting and diarrhea; some patients have respiratory symptoms without a fever. Illness with the pH1N1 virus has ranged from mild to severe. While most people who have been sick have recovered without needing medical treatment, hospitalizations and deaths from infection with this virus have occurred. Many people hospitalized with the pH1N1 virus have had one or more medical conditions previously recognized as placing people at "high risk" of serious seasonal influenza-related complications, including pregnancy, diabetes, heart disease, asthma, and kidney disease [CDC 2009a]. In contrast to seasonal influenza, nearly 90% of deaths related to pH1N1 occurred among people younger than 65 years of age [CDC 2010e].

Background on Influenza Vaccines

Vaccination is the most effective method to prevent influenza and to prevent serious illness and death from influenza infection [Cox and Subbarao 1999; Nichol and Treanor 2006]. The FDA licensed the first pH1N1 vaccine in September 2009 [FDA 2009]. Since then, the FDA approved four pH1N1 vaccines produced by four manufacturers [FDA 2009]. All of these vaccines used the same licensure and manufacturing processes as those used for the production of the seasonal influenza vaccines. The 2009 pH1N1 vaccine became available in the United States starting October 2009. The pH1N1 vaccine was available as a live, attenuated monovalent vaccine for intranasal administration and as a monovalent, inactivated, split-virus or subunit vaccine for injection [CDC 2009f].

In July 2009, the ACIP recommended that certain groups of the general population receive the 2009 pH1N1 vaccine first [CDC 2009b]. These target groups included:

- Pregnant women
- People who lived with or cared for children younger than 6 months of age
- Healthcare and emergency medical services personnel
- Persons between the ages of 6 months and 24 years old

- People aged 25–64 years who were at higher risk for 2009 pH1N1 because of chronic health disorders or compromised immune systems

The ACIP recommended that children aged 6 months–9 years receive two doses separated by approximately 4 weeks, while persons aged ≥ 10 years should receive one dose [CDC 2009g]. The live attenuated influenza nasal vaccine was recommended for use in healthy, nonpregnant persons aged 2–49 years. It was not recommended for use in children aged < 2 years, adults > 49 years, pregnant women, or persons with underlying medical conditions that confer a higher risk for influenza complications [CDC 2009g].

In two large randomized clinical trials of the immune response to the pH1N1 vaccine in 410 children and 724 adults in the United States, researchers demonstrated the efficacy of the pH1N1 vaccine. After one vaccination, 92%–100% of adults were considered to be immune [Plennevaux et al. 2010]. Studies in the United Kingdom, Australia, China, and Hungary also demonstrated the efficacy of the pH1N1 vaccine [Clark et al. 2009; Greenburg et al. 2009; Liang et al. 2010; Vajo et al. 2010].

Studies in the United States found that no deaths or vaccine-related serious adverse events occurred. Injection-site reactions (including pain, tenderness, and swelling) and systemic reactions (including fever, headache, and muscle aches) were reported, but no differences between vaccine and placebo groups occurred [Plennevaux et al. 2010].

In one published report, CDC reviewed vaccine safety results for the pH1N1 vaccines from two reports received through the U.S. VAERS and electronic data from the VSD, a large population-based database. As of November 24, 2009, VAERS data revealed 82 adverse event reports per 1 million pH1N1 vaccine doses distributed compared with 47 reports per 1 million seasonal influenza vaccine doses distributed [CDC 2009f]. No differences between pH1N1 and seasonal influenza vaccines were found in the types or proportion of serious reported adverse events. Thirteen deaths after receipt of the pH1N1 vaccine were reported. Significant underlying illness was reported in nine of these deaths, one death resulted from a motor vehicle accident, and the remaining three deaths are awaiting final review. Twelve reports of Guillain-Barre syndrome, an uncommon peripheral neuropathy that can cause paralysis and, in severe cases, respiratory failure and death, were identified by VAERS. Four of the reported cases met the official criteria for Guillain-Barre syndrome, four did not meet the criteria, and four are under review. The reported number of cases as of November 2009 was substantially smaller than the expected number for the general population. The VSD data showed no increase in monitored health events above background rates among recipients of the pH1N1 vaccine [CDC 2009f].

In another report, CDC reviewed data through March 31, 2010, from the Emerging Infections Program, which conducted active surveillance to assess the risk for Guillain-Barre syndrome after pH1N1 vaccination. These data showed that the rate of Guillain-Barre syndrome following receipt of the pH1N1 vaccine was less than one excess Guillain-Barre syndrome case per 1 million vaccinations. This is similar to the rate following the receipt of some formulations of seasonal influenza vaccines [CDC 2010f].

The 2009–2010 seasonal influenza vaccine became available in August 2009. The seasonal influenza vaccines were also available as a live, attenuated vaccine for intranasal administration and as a trivalent, inactivated vaccine for injection [CDC 2009e]. This vaccine contained three strains: A/Brisbane/59/2007 (H1N1)-like, A/Brisbane/10/2007 (H3N2)-like, and B/Brisbane 60/2008-like antigens [CDC 2009e].

In July 2009, the ACIP updated its longstanding recommendations for seasonal influenza vaccination [CDC 2009e]. The groups targeted to receive the vaccine were similar to those for the 2009 H1N1 vaccine but also included persons aged ≥ 50 years, residents of nursing homes and other long-term care facilities, and household contacts and caregivers of children aged < 5 years and adults aged ≥ 50 years, with particular emphasis on vaccinating contacts of children aged < 6 months. Target groups for both influenza vaccines included out-of-home child care providers.

The inactivated influenza injection vaccine can be used for any person aged ≥ 6 months, including those with high-risk conditions such as asthma, pregnancy, or immunosuppressive disorder. This vaccine is contraindicated and should not be administered to persons known to have anaphylactic hypersensitivity to eggs or to other components of the influenza vaccine [CDC 2010g]. The live attenuated influenza nasal vaccine may be used for healthy, nonpregnant persons aged 2–49 years [CDC 2009e].

The efficacy of influenza vaccines in adults has been shown to be 70%–90% against confirmed influenza when the vaccine strains match the circulating strains [Fukuda et al. 2004]. Influenza vaccination has also been shown to reduce the rates of influenza-like illness, lost workdays, and physician visits in healthy, working adults when the vaccine and circulating viruses are similar [Nichol et al. 1995; Bridges et al. 2000].

The inactivated influenza injection vaccine contains inactivated viruses and cannot cause influenza in vaccine recipients [CDC 2010g]. The most common side effect of seasonal influenza injection vaccines reported in adults is soreness at the injection site [Vellozzi et al. 2009]. Muscle pain, discomfort or weakness, and fever rarely occur. The live attenuated influenza nasal vaccine contains a weakened virus and cannot cause influenza in vaccine recipients. However, it can cause mild signs or symptoms including runny nose, nasal congestion, fever, or sore throat. These side effects are mild and short-lasting, especially when compared to the symptoms of seasonal influenza infection [CDC 2010g].

Child care providers are at risk of acquiring and transmitting influenza through their daily duties. Influenza can be spread quickly among children and providers in child care settings because children younger than 5 years of age are particularly vulnerable; they are constantly in close contact with one another and their providers; toys and other objects are often shared; and young children may not be able to wash their hands well or cover their mouth and nose when they cough or sneeze.

One study demonstrated the presence of influenza A virus on 23%–53% of surfaces at 14 different day care centers tested over a 6-month influenza season in 2003 [Boone and Gerba 2004]. Although incidence of influenza and other respiratory infections among child care providers is unknown, several studies have demonstrated that children attending day care are at high risk for respiratory infections [Doyle 1976; Strangert 1976; Fleming et al. 1987; Wald et al. 1988; Bell et al. 1989; Hurwitz et al. 1991].

Healthy People 2010, a national health promotion and disease prevention initiative, set the target seasonal influenza vaccination coverage rate for noninstitutionalized high-risk adults aged 18 to 64 years at 60% [US DHHS 2000]. Data regarding seasonal influenza vaccination rates among child care providers is limited. In one of two published studies on this topic, researchers found that annual seasonal influenza vaccination rates ranged from 26%–51% among child care providers at one Pennsylvania child care center between 2002 and 2007 [Lee et al. 2008]. The authors attributed an increase in vaccination rates during this study to offering free on-site vaccination. In the other study, researchers found that providing an education program increased immunization rates among child care staff at five centers from 30% in 2002 to 60% in 2003 [Hayney and Bartell 2005]. Review of the published medical literature has shown that information on knowledge of and attitudes towards influenza vaccination in this group is lacking.

ASSESSMENT

Cross-Sectional Study

We completed a cross-sectional survey of child care center employees to examine their knowledge, attitudes, and receipt of seasonal influenza and pH1N1 influenza vaccines. We also sought to determine factors that predict the likelihood of getting the vaccines.

We used the Theory of Planned Behavior [Ajzen 1991; Armitage and Conner 2001], a widely applied theory in predicting social and health behavior, in developing the questionnaire for our survey. A central factor in the Theory of Planned Behavior is that the individual's intention to perform a given behavior is predictive of actual behavior [Azjen 1991]. The Theory of Planned Behavior states that a person's attitude (positive or negative feelings towards a behavior), perception of subjective norms (the perception that there is social pressure to perform or not perform the behavior), and perceived behavioral control (the perception of choice and availability of resources necessary to perform or not perform the behavior) influence the person's intention to perform the behavior. When a person has a positive attitude towards a behavior and feels that others encourage the behavior and he or she has the choice and resources to perform the behavior, then intention to perform the behavior will typically be positive. Survey items were created to measure attitudes towards the vaccines, subjective norms regarding receiving the vaccines, and perceived behavioral control in receiving the vaccines to explore these relationships.

The questionnaire covered personal and work characteristics, pertinent medical history, and receipt of or intention to receive the pH1N1 and seasonal influenza vaccines. Demographic questions from the Behavioral Risk Factor Surveillance System Survey Questionnaire [CDC 2008] and influenza vaccine practices questions from the National 2009 H1N1 Flu Survey Questionnaire were used [CDC 2009d]. Questions drawing from the three variables of the Theory of Planned Behavior were also included to assess knowledge about and attitudes towards each vaccine [Francis et al. 2004]. Some knowledge and attitudes questions were examined by extent of agreement with statements about each vaccine, using a four-point Likert scale (i.e., disagree, somewhat disagree, somewhat agree, and agree). Other attitudes questions were examined using a four-point scale with bipolar adjectives (e.g. very good, somewhat good, somewhat bad, very bad). The questionnaire was anonymous and did not include any directly personal identifying information such as names or dates of birth.

The study population for this evaluation consisted of all employees working at randomly selected licensed child care centers in the county. All part-time and full-time employees ≥ 18 years old working at the facility on the date of our visit to the center were invited to participate. Thirty centers were selected randomly from a list of 135 licensed centers providing care to infants. An additional nine centers were selected 2 weeks later because five of the initial centers declined to participate. We contacted center directors via telephone, explained the objectives and methods of the evaluation, and invited the selected centers to participate. We set up one survey date for each center that agreed to participate.

Prior to the visit, each center director was sent an informational sheet by e-mail, fax, or mail to be distributed to employees. The informational sheet identified the purpose of the survey and when it would take place. We visited all participating child care centers from January 30– March 1, 2010. At the directors' preference, visits were made during center nap hours or during staff meetings to ensure that participation did not interfere with child care.

During and after survey administration, information about center characteristics, including center type and number of employees were collected from center directors. Additional information about center characteristics, including Step Up to Quality rating, NAEYC accreditation, and child capacity was obtained from the Ohio Department of Jobs and Family Services website [ODJFS 2010].

Data Analysis

Survey results were analyzed using descriptive statistical methods. Responses using a Likert scale were categorized as "expressed agreement" if respondents marked "agree" or "somewhat agree," and as "expressed disagreement" if respondents marked "disagree" or "somewhat disagree." Internal consistency for the attitudes, subjective norms, and perceived behavioral control variables was measured using Cronbach's coefficient (α) after adjusting for directionality. We created composite scores for variables within the attitudes, subjective norms, and perceived behavioral control domains where $\alpha > 0.7$ by calculating the mean of the individual scores for each respondent.

Characteristics of child care center employees who reported receipt of each vaccine were compared to those who denied receipt of the respective vaccine. Among those employees who denied receipt of each vaccine, characteristics of employees who reported intention to receive each vaccine were compared to those who reported no intention to receive the respective vaccine. Responses to the knowledge and attitudes questions were also compared among each group. We conducted most bivariate analyses using the Student's t-test, χ^2test, or Fisher's exact test. We used logistic regression for the bivariate analyses of the composite scores for the attitudes, subjective norms, and perceived behavioral control domains. Bivariate analyses were conducted using SPSS (SPSS Inc., Chicago, Illinois). All tests were two-tailed, and statistical significance was set at $P < 0.05$. We then used a stepwise backward elimination multiple logistic regression model to identify factors independently associated with receipt of each vaccine. The reduced stepwise logistic regression model was then analyzed using a GEE model to account for the random effect of center with SAS 9.2 (SAS Institute, Cary, North Carolina).

RESULTS

Characteristics of Participating Child Care Centers

Thirty-two (84%) of 38 invited licensed child care centers agreed to participate in the survey. One center had closed in December 2009 although its name still appeared on the list of licensed centers in operation in January 2010. The six declining centers cited lack of interest and/or lack of time as reasons for not participating. Participating and declining centers had similar characteristics (Table 1). Most participating centers were for-profit (69%) and were independent or religiously-affiliated centers (75%). Four (12%) of centers were NAEYC accredited, and 12 (38%) of centers had a Step Up to Quality rating.

Table 1. Characteristics of participating and declining child care centers

Center Characteristic	No. Participating Centers (%) n = 32	No. Declining Centers (%) n = 6
For profit	22 (69)	5 (83)
Center type		
Independent or religious affiliation	24 (75)	6 (100)
Chain or corporate or university affiliation	8 (25)	0 (0)
Number of children capacity ≥ 100	15 (47)	2 (33)
Total number of employees ≥ 15	16 (50)	3 (50)
NAEYC accredited	4 (12)	0 (0)
Has Step Up to Quality rating	12 (38)	0 (0)

Demographic and Health Characteristics of Survey Respondents

We visited all 32 participating child care centers and 384 (95%) of 403 employees ≥ 18 years old working on the day of the visits completed a survey. The median age of respondents was 30 years, with a range of 18–81 years. Most (97%) respondents were female, and 16 (4%) of responding females were pregnant at the time of the survey. The two racial groups most commonly represented were whites (52%) and blacks or African Americans (42%). Other demographic characteristics of survey respondents are shown in Table 2.

Regarding underlying medical conditions, 45 (12%) respondents reported having asthma or another chronic lung disease, 16 (4%) reported having heart disease (excluding high blood pressure), and 14 (4%) reported having diabetes. In total, 315 (82%) respondents denied having an underlying medical condition that would put them at high risk for influenza-related complications. These conditions also included kidney disease, liver disease, current diagnosis of cancer, any immunosuppressive disease, and taking immunosuppressive therapy.

Table 2. Demographic characteristics of survey respondents

Demographic Characteristic	No. Respondents (%) n = 363–384*
Female	371 (97)
Pregnant at the time of survey completion	16 (4)
Race	
Black or African American	161 (42)
White	197 (52)
Other†	23 (6)
Hispanic or Latino ethnicity	13 (4)
Household included:	
One or more adults ≥ 18 years old‡	306 (80)
One or more children ≤ 5 years old	16 (4)
One or more children 5–17 years old	204 (53)
Highest year of school completed	
High school graduate or GED or less	122 (32)
Some college or technical school or higher	262 (68)
Annual household income	
< $35,000	233 (63)
≥ $35,000	135 (37)

*Sample sizes ranged from 363–384 because of missing values.
†Other race includes those respondents who selected American Indian or Alaska Native, Asian, Native Hawaiian or Pacific Islander, or "other" for race.
‡Respondents were asked to exclude themselves when answering this question.

Work Characteristics of Survey Respondents

Most (85%) respondents were employed full time by their center. Most (62%) respondents reported caring for toddlers or children 13 months–3 years old; 25% reported caring for young infants 0–5 months; and 30% reported caring for older infants 6–12 months old. Fifty-one (13%) respondents reported not providing direct care to children. Other work characteristics are shown in Table 3.

Table 3. Work characteristics of survey respondents

Work Characteristic	No. Respondents (%) n = 384
Full-time employment	325 (85)
Median years worked in child care (range)	6 (0–50)
Median years worked at center (range)	2 (0–38)
Ages of children cared for in job*	
0–5 months	95 (25)
6–12 months	116 (30)
13 months–3 years	237 (62)
4 years and older	142 (37)
Did not provide direct care to children	51 (13)
Work at for-profit center	269 (70)
Type of center worked at	
Independent or religiously-affiliated center	252 (66)
Chain, corporate or university-affiliated center	132 (34)
Work at NAEYC accredited center	65 (17)
Work at center with Step Up to Quality rating	146 (38)

*Respondents could select more than one age group.

pH1N1 and Seasonal Influenza Vaccine Receipt, Beliefs, and Attitudes

Forty-five (12%) respondents reported having received the pH1N1 vaccine since October 2009. Rates of pH1N1 vaccination among respondents ranged from 0%–83% by child care center. Thirteen (41%) of the 32 centers had 0% pH1N1 vaccination rates among responding employees. The percentage of respondents receiving the pH1N1 vaccine by month is shown by the solid black line in Figure 1. Sixty percent of respondents who received the pH1N1 vaccine received it by November 2009. Most (96%) respondents reported receiving the pH1N1 injection vaccine rather than the nasal spray. The most common places where respondents received the pH1N1 vaccine were a doctor's office (35%) and the workplace (24%). Other places where respondents received the pH1N1 vaccine are shown in Figure 2.

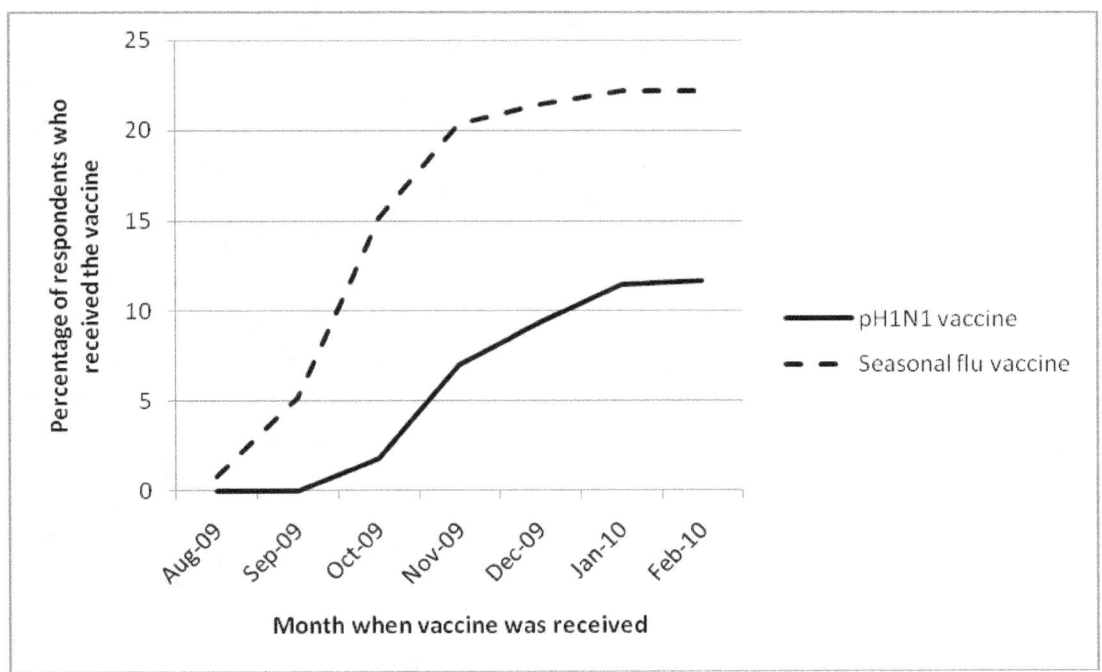

Figure 1. Month when pH1N1 and seasonal influenza vaccines were received by respondents.

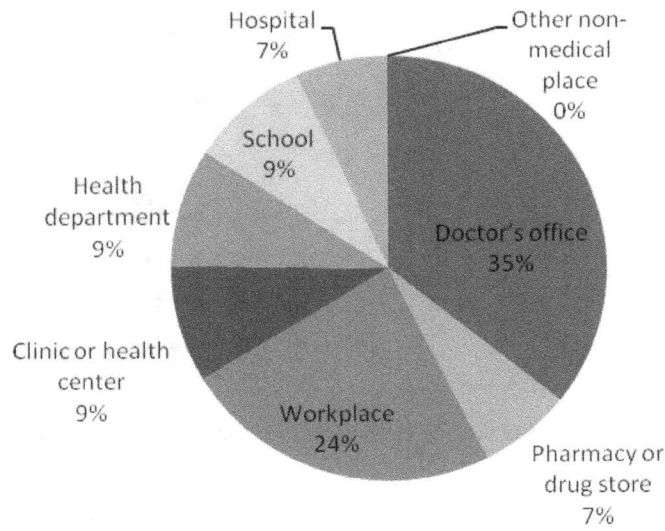

Figure 2. Pie chart displaying the locations where respondents received the pH1N1 vaccine by percentage.

Ninety-four (25%) respondents reported having received the seasonal influenza vaccine the previous year between October 2008 and April 2009. Eighty-five (22%) respondents reported having received the 2009-2010 seasonal influenza vaccine since August 2009. Rates of seasonal influenza vaccination among respondents ranged 0%–57% by child care center. Four (12%) of the 32 centers had seasonal influenza vaccination rates of 0% among responding employees. The percentage of respondents receiving the seasonal influenza vaccine by month is shown by the dashed black line in Figure 1. The majority of respondents (92%) who received the seasonal influenza vaccine received it by November 2009. Most respondents (98%) who received the seasonal influenza vaccine reported receiving the injection rather than the nasal spray. The most common places where respondents received the seasonal influenza vaccine were at a doctor's office (45%) and a pharmacy or drug store (27%). Other places where respondents received the seasonal influenza vaccine are shown in Figure 3.

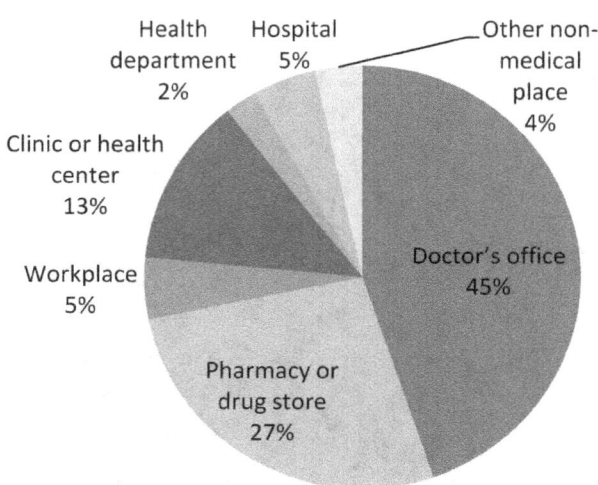

Figure 3. Pie chart displaying the locations where respondents received the seasonal influenza vaccine by percentage.

The most common reason for receiving the pH1N1 vaccine cited by respondents was protection of oneself or one's family (54%). Other reasons cited are shown in Table 4. pH1N1 vaccination rates were 14% for respondents who cared for young infants (0–5 months), 13% for those who cared for older infants (6–12 months old), 16% for those who cared for toddlers (13 months–3 years), and 11% for those who cared for children ≥ 4 years old.

The most common reason for receiving the seasonal influenza vaccine cited by respondents was to protect oneself or one's family (65%). Other reasons cited are shown in Table 4. Seasonal influenza vaccination rates were 17% for respondents who cared for young infants, 22% for those who cared for older infants, 28% for those who cared for toddlers, and 23% for those who cared for children ≥ 4 years old.

Table 4. Main reasons cited by respondents who received the pH1N1 or seasonal influenza vaccines

Main Reason Cited*	No. Respondents Who Received the pH1N1 Vaccine (%) n = 43†	No. Respondents Who Received the Seasonal Influenza Vaccine (%) n = 79‡
To protect myself/my family	23 (54)	51 (65)
My doctor recommended that I receive the vaccine	7 (16)	16 (20)
To protect the children I care for	6 (14)	5 (6)
My manager ecommended that I receive the vaccine	1 (2)	2 (3)
Other	6 (14)	5 (6)

*Respondents were asked to choose one main reason.
†Two respondents were excluded because they selected multiple reasons.
‡Six respondents were excluded because they selected multiple reasons or failed to select a reason.

Twenty-five (7%) respondents reported receiving both the pH1N1 and the seasonal influenza vaccines, 20 (5%) respondents reported receiving the pH1N1 but not the seasonal influenza vaccine, and 60 (16%) respondents reported receiving the seasonal influenza but not the pH1N1 vaccine. A total of 278 (72%) respondents reported receiving neither influenza vaccine.

Of the 339 respondents who had not received the pH1N1 influenza vaccine, 65 (19%) reported they would definitely (n = 15) or probably (n = 50) get one. In contrast, 274 (81%) reported they would definitely not (n = 127) or probably not (n = 147) get one. Of the 298 respondents who had not received the seasonal influenza vaccine, 56 (19%) reported they would definitely (n = 13) or probably (n = 43) get one. In contrast, 242 (81%) reported they would definitely not (n = 127) or probably not (n = 115) get one. One respondent did not answer this question. The most common reason cited for intending to receive either vaccine was to protect oneself or one's family. Other reasons cited are shown in Table 5. The most common reasons cited for not intending to receive either vaccine were "I don't think the vaccine will keep me from getting the flu" and "I don't think I need the vaccine." Other reasons cited are shown in Table 6.

Table 5. Reasons cited by respondents who intend to receive the pH1N1 or seasonal influenza vaccines

Reason Cited*	No. Respondents Who Intended to Receive the pH1N1 Vaccine (%) n = 65	No. Respondents Who Intended to Receive the Seasonal Influenza Vaccine (%) n = 55†
To protect myself/my family	50 (77)	38 (69)
To protect the children I care for	8 (12)	9 (16)
My doctor recommended that I receive the vaccine	3 (5)	5 (9)
My manager recommended that I receive the vaccine	0 (0)	0 (0)
Other	4 (6)	3 (6)

*Respondents were asked to choose one main reason.
†One respondent did not answer this question.

Table 6. Main reasons cited by respondents for not receiving the pH1N1 and seasonal influenza vaccines

Main Reason Cited*	No. Respondents Who Did Not Intend to Receive the pH1N1 Vaccine (%) n = 270†	No. Respondents Who Did Not Intend to Receive the Seasonal Influenza Vaccine (%) n = 235‡
I don't think I need the vaccine	67 (25)	73 (31)
I don't think the vaccine will keep me from getting the flu	43 (16)	69 (29)
The vaccine is not safe	42 (16)	13 (6)
I haven't had time to get the vaccine	16 (6)	12 (5)
It costs too much to get the vaccine	8 (3)	6 (3)
I have already had the flu	4 (2)	5 (2)
I tried to get the vaccine but could not get it	4 (2)	2 (1)
I am allergic to the vaccine	3 (1)	2 (1)
I don't know where to get the vaccine	3 (1)	2 (1)
Other	65 (24)§	43 (18)¶

*Respondents were asked to choose one main reason.
†Four respondents were excluded because they selected multiple reasons or failed to select a reason.
‡Seven respondents were excluded because they selected multiple reasons or failed to select a reason.
§The most common "other" reasons cited for not intending to receive the pH1N1 vaccine included "I don't know enough about or have enough information on the vaccine," "the vaccine is too new or was created too fast," and "I just didn't want it."
¶The most common "other" reasons cited for not intending to receive the seasonal influenza vaccine included "I just didn't want it" and "the vaccine makes me sick or gives me the flu."

Most respondents had positive attitudes towards both vaccines, as most believed both vaccines to be "beneficial," "good," and "wise" (Table 7) versus "harmful," "bad," and "unwise." These first three measures of attitudes towards the pH1N1 vaccine had a high Cronbach's (or internal consistency) coefficient of $\alpha = 0.879$. Likewise, the same measures of attitudes towards the seasonal influenza vaccine had a high Cronbach's coefficient of $\alpha = 0.865$. Thus, for subsequent analyses, we created one positive attitudes composite score for each vaccine by calculating the mean of the scores for the three items.

Table 7. Attitudes of respondents towards the pH1N1 and seasonal influenza vaccines

Quality	No. Respondents who stated that the pH1N1 vaccine is... (%) n = 374–376*	No. Respondents that stated that the seasonal influenza vaccine is... (%) n = 373–374*
Beneficial	258 (69)	304 (82)
Good	267 (71)	301 (80)
Wise	254 (68)	297 (79)

*Samples sizes varied because of missing values.

Beliefs about the pH1N1 and seasonal influenza vaccines of all respondents who answered the respective questions are shown in Table 8. Most respondents believed that transmission of both pH1N1 and seasonal influenza could occur between children and child care providers and that both types of influenza were serious infections. However, most respondents had negative beliefs about both vaccines, including that they would make them sick and that they would not prevent them from getting influenza.

Table 8. Beliefs of respondents about the pH1N1 and seasonal influenza vaccines

Belief Statement	No. Respondents Who Expressed Agreement with Statement Regarding pH1N1 (%) n = 378–383*	No. Respondents Who Expressed Agreement with Statement Regarding Seasonal Influenza (%) n = 381–382*
Child care providers can spread __ flu to children	344 (90)	359 (94)
Children can spread __ flu to child care providers	361 (95)	360 (94)
__ flu is a serious infection	345 (91)	322 (85)
The __ vaccine could make me sick	322 (84)	319 (84)
The __ vaccine will prevent me from getting the __ flu	221 (58)	213 (56)

*Sample sizes varied because of missing values.

Respondents' agreement with subjective norm statements about both vaccines is shown in Table 9. Some respondents chose not to answer specific questions; these were treated as missing values. Only one third of respondents believed that it was their duty to get either vaccine for their job. Less than half of respondents reported that their manager, doctor, or family and friends wanted them to get the vaccine, and fewer felt "social pressure" to get either vaccine. These seven subjective norms items regarding the pH1N1 vaccine had a high Cronbach's coefficient of α = 0.835. Similarly, these seven items regarding the seasonal influenza vaccine had a high Cronbach's coefficient of α = 0.839. Thus, for subsequent analyses, we created one subjective norms composite score for each vaccine by calculating the mean of the scores for the seven items.

Table 9. Agreement with subjective norm statements about the pH1N1 and seasonal influenza vaccines

Subjective Norm Statement	No. Respondents Who Expressed Agreement with Statement Regarding pH1N1 (%) n = 364–383*	No. Respondents Who Expressed Agreement with Statement Regarding Seasonal Influenza (%) n = 364–381*
It is/was my duty to get the __ vaccine for my job	116 (30)	115 (30)
A majority of my coworkers have gotten or plan to get the __ vaccine	95 (26)	128 (35)
People who are important to me want(ed) me to get the __ vaccine	115 (30)	125 (33)
My manager/employer wants(ed) me to get the __ vaccine	91 (24)	85 (23)
My doctor recommends(ed) that I get the __ vaccine	133 (35)	161 (43)
My family/friends want(ed) me to get the __ vaccine	106 (28)	121 (32)
I feel/felt social pressure to get the __ vaccine	83 (22)	63 (17)

*Sample sizes varied because of missing values.

Respondents' agreement with the perceived behavioral control statements about both vaccines is shown in Table 10. Most respondents felt that it was their decision whether or not to get each vaccine and were confident that they could get the vaccine if desired. Less than one third of respondents felt that they did not have the time or money to get the vaccine, and less than one fourth of respondents felt that getting the vaccine required a lot of effort. The latter three perceived behavioral control items regarding the pH1N1 vaccine had a high Cronbach's coefficient of α = 0.733. Similarly, the latter three items regarding the seasonal influenza vaccine had a high Cronbach's coefficient of α = 0.784. Thus, for subsequent analyses, we created one perceived behavioral control composite score for each vaccine by calculating the mean of the scores for the three items.

Table 10. Agreement with perceived behavioral control statements regarding the pH1N1 and seasonal influenza vaccines

Perceived Behavioral Control Statement	No. Respondents Who Expressed Agreement with Statement Regarding pH1N1 (%) n = 377–384*	No. Respondents Who Expressed Agreement with Statement Regarding Seasonal Influenza (%) n = 379–380*
It is/was my decision whether or not to get the __ vaccine	362 (94)	369 (97)
I am/was confident I could get the __ vaccine if I wanted	347 (91)	358 (94)
I do/did not have the time to get the __ vaccine	111 (29)	109 (29)
I do/did not have the money to get the __ vaccine	118 (31)	104 (27)
Getting the __ vaccine requires(ed) a lot of effort on my part	98 (26)	95 (25)

*Sample sizes varied because of missing values.

Factors Associated with Influenza Vaccine Receipt

We found no statistically significant associations between age, sex, or race and reporting receipt of either the pH1N1 vaccine or the seasonal influenza vaccine. However, respondents of Hispanic or Latino ethnicity were more likely to have received the pH1N1 vaccine than those not of Hispanic or Latino ethnicity (46% vs. 10%, $P < 0.01$). Hispanic or Latino ethnicity was not significantly associated with receipt of the seasonal influenza vaccine.

Annual household income and whether or not a respondent's household included adults and children ≤ 5 years old were not significantly associated with receipt of either vaccine. Respondents with children 6–17 years old in their household were more likely to get the seasonal influenza vaccine than those who did not have children 6–17 years old (29% vs. 16%, $P < 0.01$). Respondents whose highest level of education was some college or technical school or higher were more likely to have received the pH1N1 vaccine than those whose highest level of education was high school graduate or less (15% vs. 5%, $P < 0.01$). Highest level of education was not significantly associated with receipt of the seasonal influenza vaccine.

Respondents who were pregnant at the time of survey administration were more likely to have received the pH1N1 vaccine than those who were not (38% and 10%, $P < 0.01$). However, pregnancy was not associated with receipt of the seasonal influenza vaccine. Having an underlying medical condition, which includes diabetes, asthma, kidney disease, heart disease, liver disease, cancer, an immunosuppressive condition, and taking immunosuppressive therapy was not significantly associated with receipt of either vaccine.

The mean number of years worked in child care or at a particular center and whether or not a respondent provided direct care to children were not significantly associated with receipt of either vaccine. Respondents who worked part-time were more likely to have received the pH1N1 vaccine than those who worked full-time (24% vs. 10%, $P < 0.01$). Respondents who cared for toddlers (aged 13 months–3 years) were also more likely to have received the pH1N1 vaccine than those who did not (16% vs. 5%, $P < 0.01$). Respondents who cared for young infants (aged 0–5 months) were less likely to have received the seasonal influenza vaccine than those who did not (14% vs. 25%, $P < 0.01$). The other age groups of children cared for among respondents were not significantly associated with receipt of either vaccine.

Respondents who worked at corporate or university-affiliated or chain child care centers were more likely to have received the pH1N1 vaccine (22% vs. 6%, $P < 0.01$) and the seasonal influenza vaccine (29% vs. 19%, $P = 0.02$) compared to those who worked at independent or religiously-affiliated centers. Respondents who worked at NAEYC-accredited centers were more likely to have received the pH1N1 vaccine than those who worked at nonaccredited centers (28% vs. 8%, $P < 0.01$). The other center characteristics, including nonprofit status, total children and employees, and Step Up to Quality rating, were not significantly associated with reporting receipt of either vaccine.

Respondents who believed in the efficacy of the pH1N1 vaccine were more likely to have received the vaccine than those who did not believe (17% vs. 4%, $P < 0.01$). Expressing agreement with the other belief statements in Table 8 was not significantly associated with receipt of the pH1N1 vaccine. Respondents who believed in the efficacy of the seasonal influenza vaccine were more likely to have received the vaccine than those who did not believe (33% vs. 8%, $P < 0.01$) in its efficacy. Respondents who believed that the seasonal influenza vaccine could make them sick were also less likely to have received the vaccine than those who did not (20% vs. 34%, $P = 0.01$). Expressing agreement with the other belief statements in Table 8 was not significantly associated with receipt of the seasonal influenza vaccine.

Respondents with a higher positive attitudes composite score for the pH1N1 and seasonal influenza vaccines, or those who had more positive attitudes towards the vaccines were more likely to have received that vaccine ($P < 0.01$ for both vaccines). Respondents with a higher subjective norms composite score for the pH1N1 vaccine and the seasonal influenza vaccine, or those who felt external pressure from others to receive the vaccine were more likely to have received that vaccine ($P < 0.01$ for both vaccines). In addition, respondents with a higher perceived behavioral control composite score for the pH1N1 vaccine and the seasonal influenza vaccine, or those who felt personal control over whether or not to get the vaccine were more likely to have received that vaccine ($P = 0.04$ for the pH1N1 vaccine and $P = 0.02$ for the seasonal influenza vaccine).

Variables with $P < 0.05$ that were associated with receipt of the pH1N1 vaccine were selected and entered into a stepwise backward elimination multiple logistic regression model and then a GEE model to determine which ones were independently associated with receipt of the vaccine (Table 11). Factors independently associated with receipt of the pH1N1 vaccine included having some college or technical school or higher be the highest level of education ($P < 0.01$), caring for toddlers ($P = 0.03$), having positive attitudes towards the vaccine ($P < 0.01$), feeling external pressure to get the vaccine ($P < 0.01$), and feeling personal control over whether or not to get the vaccine ($P = 0.04$).

Table 11. Variables associated with receipt of the pH1N1 vaccine entered into stepwise logistic regression model

Variable	P value
Some college or higher as highest level of education	<0.01
Full-time employment	Not significant
Caring for children 13 months–3 months (toddlers)	0.03
Working at a chain, corporate or university-affiliated center	Not significant
Believing in the efficacy of the pH1N1 vaccine	Not significant
Positive attitudes composite score (i.e., having positive attitudes towards the pH1N1 vaccine)	<0.01
Subjective norms composite score (i.e., feeling external pressure to get the pH1N1 vaccine)	<0.01
Perceived behavioral control composite score (i.e., feeling personal control over whether or not to get the pH1N1 vaccine)	0.04

Variables with $P < 0.05$ that were associated with receipt of the seasonal influenza vaccine were selected and entered into a stepwise backward elimination multiple logistic regression model and then a GEE model to determine which ones were independently associated with receipt of the vaccine (Table 12). Factors independently associated with receipt of the seasonal influenza vaccine included believing in the efficacy of the seasonal influenza vaccine ($P < 0.01$), having positive attitudes towards the vaccine ($P < 0.01$), feeling external pressure to get the vaccine ($P < 0.01$), and feeling personal control over whether or not to get the vaccine ($P = 0.03$). Caring for young infants ($P = 0.02$) and having children 6–17 years old in the household ($P < 0.01$) were independently associated with not receiving the vaccine.

Table 12. Variables associated with receipt of the seasonal influenza vaccine entered into stepwise logistic regression model

Variable	P value
Not having children 6–17 years in the household	<0.01
Not caring for children 0–5 months (young infants)	0.02
Working at a chain, corporate or university-affiliated center	Not significant
Believing in the efficacy of the seasonal influenza vaccine	<0.01
Believing that the seasonal influenza vaccine could make them sick	Not significant
Positive attitudes composite score (i.e., having positive attitudes towards the seasonal influenza vaccine)	<0.01
Subjective norms composite score (i.e., feeling external pressure to get the seasonal influenza vaccine)	<0.01
Perceived behavioral control composite score (i.e., feeling personal control over whether or not to get the seasonal influenza vaccine)	0.03

Factors Associated with Intention to Receive the Influenza Vaccines

Among those respondents who reported they had not received the pH1N1 vaccine (n = 339), those who reported Hispanic or Latino ethnicity (57% vs. 18%, $P < 0.01$) and caring for toddlers aged 13 months–3 years (23% vs. 14%, $P = 0.03$) were more likely to report intention to receive the vaccine that those without these characteristics. In addition, those who reported believing that pH1N1 infection is a serious infection (21% vs. 0%, $P < 0.01$), believing in the efficacy of the vaccine (26% vs. 11%, $P < 0.01$), and believing that the pH1N1 vaccine could make them sick (33% vs. 17%, $P < 0.01$) were more likely to report intention to receive the vaccine than those without these beliefs. Similar to those that received the pH1N1 vaccine, those who reported having positive attitudes towards the vaccine ($P < 0.01$), feeling external pressure to get the vaccine ($P < 0.01$), and feeling personal control over whether or not to get the vaccine ($P < 0.01$) were more likely to have reported intention to receive the pH1N1 vaccine than those not reporting this.

Variables with $P < 0.05$ that were associated with intention to receive the pH1N1 vaccine were selected and entered into a stepwise backward elimination multiple logistic regression model and then a GEE model to determine which ones were independently associated with intention to receive the vaccine (Table 13). Factors independently associated with intention to receive the pH1N1 vaccine included caring for toddlers ($P = 0.02$), having positive attitudes towards the vaccine ($P < 0.01$), and feeling external pressure to get the vaccine ($P < 0.01$).

Table 13. Variables associated with intention to receive the pH1N1 vaccine entered into stepwise logistic regression model

Variable	P value
Caring for children 13 months–3 months (toddlers)	0.02
Believing that pH1N1 is a serious infection	Not significant
Believing in the efficacy of the pH1N1 vaccine	Not significant
Believing that the pH1N1 vaccine could make them sick	Not significant
Positive attitudes composite score (i.e., having positive attitudes towards the pH1N1 vaccine)	<0.01
Subjective norms composite score (i.e., feeling external pressure to get the pH1N1 vaccine)	<0.01
Perceived behavioral control composite score (i.e., feeling personal control over whether or not to get the pH1N1 vaccine)	Not significant

Among those who reported they had not received the seasonal influenza vaccine (n = 297), those who reported Hispanic or Latino ethnicity (62% vs. 17%, $P < 0.01$) and an annual household income of less than $35,000 (23% vs. 10%, $P < 0.01$) were more likely to have reported intention to receive the seasonal influenza vaccine than those without these characteristics. In addition, those who reported believing in the efficacy of the seasonal influenza vaccine (28% vs. 10%, $P < 0.01$), having positive attitudes towards the vaccine ($P < 0.01$), and feeling external pressure from other to receive the vaccine ($P < 0.01$) were more likely to have reported intention to receive the seasonal influenza vaccine than those without these beliefs and attitudes.

Variables with $P < 0.05$ that were associated with intention to receive the seasonal influenza vaccine were selected and entered into a stepwise backward elimination multiple logistic regression model and then a GEE model to determine which ones were independently associated with intention to receive the vaccine (Table 14). Factors independently associated with intention to receive the seasonal influenza vaccine included having an annual household income < $35,000 ($P < 0.01$), having positive attitudes towards the vaccine ($P < 0.01$), and feeling external pressure to get the vaccine ($P < 0.01$).

Table 14. Variables associated with intention to receive the seasonal influenza vaccine entered into stepwise logistic regression model

Variable	P value
Annual household income < $35,000	<0.01
Believing in the efficacy of the seasonal influenza vaccine	Not significant
Positive attitudes composite score (i.e., having positive attitudes towards the seasonal influenza vaccine)	<0.01
Subjective norms composite score (i.e., feeling external pressure to get the seasonal influenza vaccine)	<0.01

DISCUSSION

Only 12% of responding child care center employees reported having received the pH1N1 vaccine since October 2009, and only 22% reported having received the seasonal influenza vaccine since August 2009. CDC's ACIP initially recommended that caregivers for children younger than 6 months of age be included in the initial target group to receive the pH1N1 vaccine because young infants are at high risk for influenza complications, but influenza vaccines are not approved for children under 6 months old [CDC 2009d]. Despite these recommendations, only 14% of child care center employees caring for children 0–5 months received the pH1N1 vaccine. CDC's 2009 ACIP recommendations include caregivers of children aged < 5 years in the target group for seasonal influenza vaccination [CDC 2009f]. Despite these recommendations, only 22% of child care center employees reported having received the seasonal influenza vaccine. This is well below the target vaccine rate of 60% for noninstitutionalized adults set forth by Healthy People 2010 [US DHHS 2000]. These findings demonstrate that vaccine promotion in this occupational group needs improvement.

No published studies regarding pH1N1 vaccination in child care center employees exist to date, and data regarding seasonal influenza vaccination rates among this group is limited. Our pH1N1 and seasonal influenza vaccine rates were lower than the seasonal influenza vaccine rates found by Lee and colleagues (26%–51% among child care providers at one Pennsylvania child care center between 2002 and 2007) [Lee et al. 2008]. In that study, the 51% vaccine coverage rate occurred during the year that free on-site vaccination was offered. Two thirds of those who were vaccinated indicated that they would not have been vaccinated without the intervention, and one third stated they would not have been vaccinated if they needed to pay for it. Other studies have also shown that offering free vaccines to healthcare personnel leads to higher coverage rates [Ohrt and McKinney 1992; Thomas et al. 1993; Nafziger and Herwaldt 1994; Nichol and Hauge 1997; Hall et al. 1998; Martinello et al. 2003].

Our vaccine rates were also lower than those found by Hayney and Bartell (30%–60% among child care staff at five centers in Wisconsin between 2002 and 2003) [Hayney and Bartell 2005]. In that study, the 60% rate occurred the year the authors conducted an education program as part of a regular staff or education meeting at each center. Findings from this study demonstrate that offering free on-site influenza vaccination and a vaccination education program as part of regular staff meetings may significantly increase vaccination rates in child care employees.

The vaccine rates of 12% for pH1N1 and 22% for seasonal influenza in our group of child care center employees are lower than those estimated by a national study of healthcare personnel, another group targeted for vaccination, (37% for pH1N1 and 62% for seasonal influenza) as of mid-January 2010 [CDC 2010b]. The 12% pH1N1 vaccine rate among our group of child care center employees was also lower than that estimated for persons ≥ 18 years in the state of Ohio, which was 18% [CDC 2010c]. The 22% seasonal influenza vaccine rate among our group of child care center employees was also lower than that estimated for persons ≥ 18 years in the state of Ohio, which was 41% [CDC 2010d]. Because survey administration for this evaluation occurred in February, the discrepancy in vaccine rates between our child care center employees and the general adult population may be even greater. This discrepancy demonstrates the need for targeted marketing promoting influenza vaccination in this occupational group.

The most common main reason cited for receiving the pH1N1 and seasonal influenza vaccines were to protect oneself and one's family. The most common main reasons cited for not receiving the pH1N1 and seasonal influenza vaccine were "I don't think I need the vaccine," "I don't think the vaccine will keep me from getting the flu," and "the vaccine is not safe." This suggests that the three major barriers to receiving either vaccine include that many child care employees do not believe themselves to be at risk for influenza, many do not think that the vaccine is effective, and many do not think the vaccine is safe.

These cited reasons are similar to those most commonly cited by respondents of a community study examining intent to receive the pH1N1 vaccine. These included the belief that they were unlikely to be infected, concern over vaccine side effects, and a perception that if infected the illness would be mild [CDC 2009c]. The most frequently cited reasons for nonvaccination with either vaccine among surveyed healthcare personnel in the national study were "I don't need it" and "I may experience side effects" [CDC 2010b]. Concern about adverse reactions was the most common primary reason cited for not getting the seasonal influenza vaccine among registered nurses in one U.S. study [Clark et al. 2009]. Thus, these barriers are not exclusive to child care employees and are present in healthcare personnel and the general population.

More than 90% of respondents expressed agreement that child care providers and children can spread each influenza infection amongst each other and more than 80% of respondents expressed agreement that each influenza infection is serious. However, 25% and 31% of respondents cited "I don't think I need the vaccine" as the main reason for not receiving the pH1N1 and seasonal influenza vaccines, respectively. This lack of perceived need has also been shown to be a common reason for influenza vaccine refusal in healthcare personnel [Norton et al. 2008] and should be addressed in vaccine promotion efforts.

Sixteen percent of respondents selected "I don't think the pH1N1 vaccine will keep me from getting the pH1N1 flu," and 29% of respondents selected "I don't think the seasonal influenza vaccine will keep me from getting the seasonal flu," as the main reason for not getting each vaccine. However, 42% and 44% of respondents believed that the pH1N1 and seasonal influenza vaccines would not prevent them from getting the respective influenza infection. Thus, almost half of respondents doubt the efficacy of both vaccines. In addition, 84% of respondents believed that each vaccine "could make me sick" though influenza vaccination cannot cause influenza [CDC 2010g]. Belief in these commonly held influenza vaccine misconceptions was also found to be associated with influenza vaccine declination among healthcare personnel in other U.S. studies [Heimberger et al. 1995; Nichol and Hauge 1997; Martinello et al. 2003; LaVela et al. 2004; Nowalk et al. 2008; Hollmeyer et al. 2009].

Both the health departments of the county and the city held free vaccine clinics for residents throughout the winter. Despite this, almost one third of respondents felt that they did not have the money to get the pH1N1 and seasonal influenza vaccines, which suggests that these offerings were not widely known. Public health messages should emphasize that the vaccine will be offered at no cost when appropriate.

While pregnancy was significantly associated with receipt of each vaccine, reporting other medical conditions associated with a high risk of serious seasonal influenza-related complications was not. These conditions include diabetes; asthma; cancer; immunosuppressive conditions; and kidney, heart, and liver disease. This suggests that public health messages targeting vaccine promotion in these high risk groups may have been ineffective.

Our bivariate analyses revealed that employees working at corporate or university-affiliated child care centers and at chain child care centers were more likely to have received the pH1N1 vaccine. Eleven (24%) of 45 respondents who received the pH1N1 vaccine reported receiving it at the workplace. Ten of these 11 respondents worked for the same university-affiliated child care center. This center had the highest pH1N1 vaccine rate of all of the centers at 83%, and 92% of respondents from this center expressed agreement that their manager/employer wanted them to get the pH1N1 vaccine. Thus, employer recommendations to obtain the vaccine and employer facilitation of receipt of the vaccine at the workplace seems to have greatly influenced vaccination rates among employees at this center. Employer requirement of influenza vaccine has been shown to be associated with higher rates of pH1N1 and seasonal influenza vaccination among healthcare personnel [CDC 2010b].

We found that self-reported pH1N1 vaccine rates (12%) were lower than those for seasonal influenza (22%) in child care center employees. Because the pH1N1 vaccine was not available before October 2009, this may have contributed to low vaccination levels among this group. In addition, respondents who reported no intention of receiving the pH1N1 cited reasons including, "I don't know enough about or have enough information on the vaccine" and "the vaccine is too new or was created too fast," as additional reasons not to get the vaccine. These are reasons unique to the pH1N1 vaccine and were likely a major reason why the pH1N1 vaccine rate was lower than the seasonal influenza vaccine rate in this group.

Factors independently associated with receipt of each vaccine included having positive attitudes towards the vaccine, feeling external pressure to get vaccinated, and feeling personal control over whether or not to get the vaccine. These findings suggest that employees' feelings towards the vaccines and perceptions about getting the vaccines were more predictive of receipt of each vaccine than demographic and work characteristics and underlying medical conditions. Perception of external pressure from managers and coworkers likely played a contributory role in the 13 centers that had 0% pH1N1 vaccination rates and 4 centers that had 0% seasonal influenza vaccination rates among employees.

Having positive attitudes towards the vaccines and feeling external pressure to get vaccinated were also independently associated with intention to receive each vaccine. Since perceiving pressure to get the vaccine from various sources was associated with receipt of and intention to receive each vaccine, physicians and employers should improve efforts to recommend influenza vaccination for child care center employees. Since less than one third of respondents felt it was their duty to get either vaccine for their job, public health messages emphasizing personal responsibility may also be effective.

Our evaluation was subject to some limitations. First, respondents self-reported their receipt of either vaccine, and this may have been subject to recall bias. Vaccination was not validated by medical records, and respondents may have confused receipt of the pH1N1 and seasonal influenza vaccinations. Second, because the survey period was in early 2010 when pH1N1 and seasonal influenza vaccines were widely available, the accuracy of respondents' intention to receive either vaccine is uncertain. Selection bias was not likely a limitation given our high participation rate of 95%.

CONCLUSIONS

Employees at child care centers in the county had low rates of pH1N1 and seasonal influenza vaccination. Factors associated with receipt of either vaccine included having positive attitudes towards the vaccine and feeling external pressure from others to get the vaccine. Misconceptions about the need for the vaccines and the efficacy and safety of the vaccines were the most common reasons cited for not receiving either vaccine. Efforts to improve vaccination rates among this occupational group should focus on eliminating the identified barriers and addressing antivaccination ideas.

RECOMMENDATIONS

A comprehensive strategy to prevent the spread of influenza in child care centers should include all of the following: vaccination of children and providers, hand hygiene, respiratory etiquette, observing children for symptoms of respiratory illness, and encouraging sick children and employees to stay home. Vaccination is a pivotal part of this comprehensive strategy and is the most effective method to prevent serious illness and death from influenza infection [Cox and Subbarao 1999; Nichol and Treanor 2006]. Vaccination has been shown to reduce illness and absenteeism caused by influenza. Child care center employees should receive influenza vaccination to protect themselves, their families, and the children whom they care for from influenza. Annual influenza vaccination is now recommended for all persons aged ≥ 6 months who do not have contraindications to vaccination for the 2010–2011 influenza season [CDC 2010g]. The 2010–2011 trivalent vaccines will protect against pH1N1 and two other influenza viruses [CDC 2010g].

The three key phases to a successful vaccination campaign are notification, education, and vaccination [Hofmann et al. 2006]. Based on our findings, we recommend actions corresponding to these key phases and list them below to increase influenza vaccination rates among employees at child care centers.

Recommendations for the County Department of Jobs and Family Services and County Public Health

1. Keep child care center employees and the general population informed of vaccination campaigns through television spots, local newspapers, radio stations, Internet postings, mass e-mails, and social networking sites. A community assessment conducted in North Carolina showed that knowledge about the pH1N1 vaccine was obtained from multiple sources: television (85%), newspapers (52%), radio (46%), the Internet (36%), and family or friends (35%) [CDC 2009c]. Communication through local newspapers, flyers, billboards, internet posting, radio station updates, television spots, and mass e-mailing also proved to be effective during the pH1N1 vaccination campaign in Skokie, Illinois [CDC 2010h]. Free influenza materials in print form, Web tools, badges and buttons, and video/audio tools can be downloaded from CDC at http://www.cdc.gov/flu/freeresources/.

2. Address the most frequent antivaccination ideas in public health messages. Such concepts include the perceived low risk for infection, perceived lack of vaccine efficacy, and lack of knowledge of vaccine safety. Messages should address these issues and emphasize that the vaccine is offered at no cost by the county at various locations. Develop targeted messages for child care employees about their job-associated risks of infection and the importance of vaccination in keeping themselves, their families, the children they care for, and their coworkers healthy.

3. Continue to offer free training and consultation services to child care centers by the Healthy Child Care Ohio program through the county Public Health. These services should also be advertised by the county Department of Jobs and Family Services to ensure that centers are aware of available resources. Consider offering more specific training on influenza to child care center employees. Training should educate child care employees about their risk for infection and severe illness as well as the efficacy and safety of the vaccine. Misconceptions about influenza and the vaccine should be debunked. Educational messages should emphasize that child care providers have a responsibility to themselves, their families, the children they care for, and

their coworkers to get vaccinated. An education program focusing on information about vaccine-preventable diseases as part of a regular staff or education meeting was thought to be effective in increasing seasonal influenza vaccination rates in five centers in Wisconsin [Hayney and Bartell 2005].

4. Consider offering alternative education programs to those referenced in recommendation 3, which may consist of off-site seminars, educational films, informational sheets, or e-mail communications. These programs should include the components listed in the above recommendation.

5. Consider partnering to make influenza vaccination available and free at child care centers. Vaccinations should be offered to both staff members and to children. Almost one third of our surveyed child care center employees felt that they did not have the time to get either vaccine. Targeting this group by setting up vaccination clinics at 13 child care facilities proved to be effective during the pH1N1 vaccination campaign in Skokie, Illinois [CDC 2010h].

6. Emphasize the importance of influenza vaccination among pregnant women and individuals with high-risk medical conditions in public health messages and in educational programs. These groups are at highest risk for developing influenza-related complications [CDC 2010e].

7. Emphasize the importance of influenza vaccination among employees who care for children 0–5 months old in public health messages and in educational programs. Young infants are at high risk for influenza complications, but the influenza vaccines are not approved for children under 6 months old. Therefore, it is essential that those who provide care to young infants to get vaccinated to reduce the risk of influenza transmission.

Recommendations for Child Care Center Employers and Directors

1. Recommend the influenza vaccine to all employees, especially among employees who care for children 0–5 months old. Young infants are at high risk for influenza complications, but the influenza vaccines are not approved for children under 6 months old. Encourage employees to get vaccinated by including messages in e-mails, center

RECOMMENDATIONS
(CONTINUED)

newsletters, and enclosed in paychecks. Messages should be encouraging and highlight motivators such as protecting family members and the children for whom employees care. Suggested messages are "To protect the health of our children, as well as yourself and your family, it's recommended that you get a flu shot," and "Our children and families thank you for helping to keep the flu out of [facility name]. Get vaccinated!" or "Protect yourself, the children you care for, and your family from the flu by getting vaccinated!"

2. Take advantage of the free training and consultation services to child care centers offered by the county Public Health. This program is a partnership between the Ohio Department of Health and the Ohio Child Care Resource and Referral Association. A public health nurse serves as a Child Care Health Consultant and can provide free advice and training on a wide range of topics that includes immunizations and communicable diseases. More information about these services can be found by calling (513) 946-7881 or by going to the county Public Health website at http://www.hamiltoncountyhealth.org/en/programs_and_services/community_health_services/daycare_centers.html.

3. Obtain up-to-date information on clinics that offer the influenza vaccine, encourage your employees to obtain it, and share the information with them through e-mail, center newsletters, or informational sheets.

4. Identify an employee who can advocate for the receipt of the influenza vaccine to coworkers. Provide this employee "champion" with information regarding the benefits of influenza vaccination, and encourage this employee "champion" to share this information throughout the workplace. This has been shown to be effective in increasing influenza vaccination rates among healthcare personnel [Slaunwhite et al. 2009].

5. Develop an employee-management committee to explore creating a policy requiring employees to get the influenza vaccine as part of a comprehensive influenza prevention strategy. Implementing this requirement has been demonstrated to be effective among healthcare personnel [CDC 2010b].

RECOMMENDATIONS
(CONTINUED)

6. Develop an employee-management committee to explore the feasibility of offering seasonal influenza vaccination to employees at your child care center. The center with the highest pH1N1 vaccination rate of 83% in our evaluation offered the vaccine at the workplace. Offer the vaccine to employees at no cost whenever possible since almost one third of respondents in our evaluation felt that they did not have the money to get either vaccine. Consider partnering with the local health department or local healthcare providers.

7. Consider offering incentives to employees who get vaccinated. Suggestions include raffles of a "free" day off or gift cards. Attempts to create friendly competition among rooms to achieve the highest rates can be considered, and the winner could be rewarded with a prize such as a free lunch.

8. Obtain more information on other ways to prevent the spread of influenza at child care centers at http://www.cdc.gov/flu/professionals/infectioncontrol/childcaresettings.htm /.

Recommendations for Child Care Center Employees

1. Get the seasonal influenza vaccine every year. The county Public Health is offering the 2010–2011 seasonal influenza vaccine free of charge at various health clinics and community centers throughout the county. Vaccination locations can be found by going to the county Public Health flu shot location website at http://www.hamiltoncountyhealth.org/resourceSearch.aspx?publish=1&lang=en&type=4 or by calling (513) 931-SHOT. Additional information for flu shot providers nationwide can be found at http://www.flucliniclocator.org/.

2. Stay informed. Obtain information about influenza and the influenza vaccine from reliable sources. The National Library of Medicine and the National Institutes of Health offer guidelines for evaluating the quality of health information at http://www.nlm.nih.gov/medlineplus/evaluatinghealthinformation.html.

RECOMMENDATIONS
(CONTINUED)

3. Discuss other options for preventing influenza with your healthcare provider if you have any contraindications to receiving either the influenza injection or nasal vaccine.

4. Be an influenza vaccine "champion," and encourage your coworkers to get the influenza vaccine.

5. Obtain more information on other ways to protect yourselves and prevent the spread of influenza at child care centers at http://www.cdc.gov/flu/school/.

REFERENCES

Armitage CJ, Conner M [2001]. Efficacy of the theory of planned behaviour: a metaanalytic review. Br J Soc Psychol 40(Pt 4):471–499.

Azjen I [1991]. The theory of planned behavior. Organ Behav Hum Decis Process 50(2):179–211.

Bell DM, Gleiber DW, Mercer AA, Phifer R, Guinter RH, Cohen AJ, Epstein EU, Narayanan M [1989]. Illness associated with childcare: a study of incidence and cost. Am J Public Health 79(4):479–484.

Blachere FM, Lindsley WG, Pearce TA, Anderson SE, Fisher M, Khakoo R, Meade BJ, Lander O, Davis S, Thewlis RE, Celik I, Chen BT, Beezhold DH [2009]. Measurement of airborne influenza virus in a hospital emergency department. Clin Infect Dis 48(15):438–440.

Boone SA, Gerba CP [2004]. The occurrence of influenza A virus on household and day care center fomites. J Infect 51(2):103–109.

Bridges CB, Kuehnert MJ, Hall CB [2003]. Transmission of influenza: implications for control in health care settings. Clin Infect Dis 37(8):1094–1101.

Bridges CB, Thompson WW, Martin MI, Reeve GR, Talamonti WJ, Cox NJ, Lilac HA, Hall H, Klimov A, Fujuda K [2000]. Effectiveness and cost-benefit of influenza vaccination of health working adults: a randomized controlled trial. JAMA 284(13):1655–1663.

CDC (Centers for Disease Control and Prevention) [2008]. Behavioral Risk Factor Surveillance System Survey Questionnaire. Atlanta, Georgia: U.S. Department of Health and Human Services, Centers for Disease Control and Prevention.

CDC [2009a]. 2009 H1N1 Flu ("Swine Flu") and You. [http://www.cdc.gov/H1N1flu/qa.htm]. Date accessed: September 2010.

CDC [2009b]. 2009 H1N1 Vaccination Recommendations. [http://www.cdc.gov/h1n1flu/vaccination/acip.htm]. Date accessed: September 2010.

REFERENCES
(CONTINUED)

CDC [2009c]. Intent to receive influenza A (H1N1) 2009 monovalent and seasonal influenza vaccines – Two Counties, North Carolina, August 2009. MMWR 58(50):1401–1404.

CDC [2009d]. National 2009 H1N1 Flu Survey Questionnaire. Atlanta, Georgia: U.S. Department of Health and Human Services, Centers for Disease Control and Prevention.

CDC [2009e]. Prevention and Control of Seasonal Influenza with Vaccines: Recommendations of the Advisory Committee on Immunization Practices (ACIP). MMWR 58(RR-8):1–52.

CDC [2009f]. Safety of influenza A (H1N1) 2009 monovalent vaccines - United States, October 1–November 24, 2009. MMWR 58(48):1351–1356.

CDC [2009g]. Update on Influenza A (H1N1) 2009 monovalent vaccines. MMWR 58(39):1100–1101.

CDC [2010a]. Estimates of deaths associated with seasonal influenza – United States, 1976-2007. MMWR 59(33):1057–1062.

CDC [2010b]. Interim results: influenza A (H1N1) 2009 monovalent and seasonal influenza vaccination coverage among health-care personnel – United States, August 2009–January 2010. MMWR 59(12):357–362.

CDC [2010c]. Interim results: state-specific influenza A (H1N1) 2009 monovalent vaccination coverage – United States, October 2009–January 2010. MMWR 59(12):363–368.

CDC [2010d]. Interim results: state-specific seasonal influenza vaccination coverage – United States, October 2009–January 2010. MMWR 59(16):477–484.

CDC [2010e]. Key Facts About Influenza (Flu) & Flu Vaccine. [http://www.cdc.gov/flu/keyfacts.htm]. Date accessed: September 2010.

CDC [2010f]. Preliminary results: surveillance for Guillain-Barre syndrome after receipt of influenza A (H1N1) 2009 monovalent vaccine – United States, 2009-2010. MMWR 59(21):657–661.

CDC [2010g]. Prevention and Control of Influenza with Vaccines: Recommendations of the Advisory Committee on Immunization Practices (ACIP). MMWR 59(No. RR-8):1–62.

CDC [2010h]. Regional Influenza A (H1N1) 2009 monovalent vaccination campaign – Skokie, Illinois, October 16– December 31, 2009. MMWR 59(29):909–913.

CDC [2010i]. Updated CDC Estimates of 2009 H1N1 Influenza Cases, Hospitalizations and Deaths in the United States, April 2009–April 10, 2010. [http://www.cdc.gov/h1n1flu/estimates_2009_h1n1.htm]. Date accessed: September 2010.

Clark SJ, Cowan AE, Wortley PM [2009]. Influenza vaccination attitudes and practices among US registered nurses. Am J Infect Control 2009 37(7):551–556.

Cox NJ, Subbarao K [1999]. Influenza. Lancet 354(9186):1277–1282.

Doyle A [1976]. Incidence of illness in early group and family day care. Pediatrics 58(4):607–612.

Fleming DW, Cochi SL, Hightower AW, Broome CV [1987]. Childhood upper respiratory tract infections: to what degree is incidence affected by day care attendance? Pediatrics 79(1):55–60.

Food and Drug Administration [2009]. Influenza A (H1N1) 2009 monovalent. [http://www.fda.gov/biologicsbloodvaccines/vaccines/approvedproducts/ucm181950.htm]. Date accessed: October 2010.

Francis JJ, Eccles MP, Johnston M, Walker A, Grimshaw J, Foy R, Kaner EFS, Zmith L, Bonetti D [2004]. Constructing questionnaires based on the theory of planned behavior: a manual for health services researchers. University of Newcastle Upon Tyne: Centre for Health Services Research edition. University of Newcastle Upon Tyne.

Fukuda K, Levandowski RA, Bridges CB, Cox NJ [2004]. Inactivated influenza vaccines. In: Plotkin SA, Orenstein WA, eds. Vaccines. 4th ed. Philadelphia, PA: Saunders, pp. 339–370.

REFERENCES
(CONTINUED)

Greenberg ME, Lai MH, Hartel GF, Wichems CH, Gittleson C, Bennet J, Dawson G, Hu W, Leggio C, Washington D, Basser RL [2009]. Response to a monovalent 2009 influenza A (H1N1) vaccine. N Engl J Med 361(25):2405-2413.

Hall KL, Holmes SS, Evans, ME [1998]. Increasing hospital employee participation in an influenza vaccine program. Am J Infect Control 26(9):367-368.

Hayney MS, Bartell JC [2005]. An immunization education program for childcare providers. J School Health 75(4):147-150.

Heimberger T, Chang HG, Shaikh M, Crotty L, Morse D, Birkhead G [1995]. Knowledge and attitudes of healthcare workers about influenza: why are they not getting vaccinated? Infect Control Hosp Epidemiol 16(7):412-415.

Hofmann F, Ferracin C, Marsh, G, Dumas R [2006]. Influenza vaccination of healthcare workers: a literature review of attitudes and beliefs. Infection 34(3):142-147.

Hollmeyer HG, Hayden F, Poland G, Buchholz U [2009]. Influenza vaccination of health care workers in hospitals—a review of studies on attitudes and predictors. Vaccine 27(30):3935-3944.

Hurwitz ES, Gunn WJ, Pinsky PF, Schonberger LB [1991]. Risk of respiratory illness associated with day care attendance: a nationwide study. Pediatrics 87(1):62-29.

LaVela SL, Smith B, Weaver FM, Legro MW, Goldstein B, Nichol K [2004]. Attitudes and practices regarding influenza vaccination among healthcare workers providing services to individuals with spinal cord injuries and siorders. Infect Control Hosp Epidemiol 25(11):933-940.

Lee I, Thompson S, Lautenbach E, Gasink LB, Watson B, Fishman NO, Chen Z, Linkin DR [2008]. Effect of accessibility of influenza vaccination on the rate of childcare staff vaccination. Infect Control Hosp Epidemiol 29(5):465-467.

Liang XF, Wang HQ, Fang HH, Wu J, Zhu FC, Li RC, Xia SL, Zhao YL, Li FJ, Yan SH, Yin WD, An K, Feng DJ, Cui CL, Qi FC, Ju CJ, Zhang YH, Guo ZJ, Chen PY, Chen Z, Yan KM, Wang Y [2010]. Safety and immunogenicity of 2009 pandemic influenza A

REFERENCES
(CONTINUED)

H1N1 vaccines in China: a multicentre, double-blind, randomised, placebo-controlled trial. Lancet 375(9708):56–66.

Lindsley WG, Blachere FM, Davis KA, Pearce TA, Fisher MA, Khakoo R, Davis SM, Rogers ME, Thewlis RE, Posada JA, Redrow JB, Celik IB, Chen BT, Beezhold DH [2010a]. Distribution of airborne influenza virus and respiratory syncytial virus in an urgent care medical clinic. Clin Infect Dis 50(5):693–8.

Lindsley WG, Blachere FM, Thewlis RE, Vishnu A, Davis KA, Cao G, Palmer JE, Clark KE, Fisher MA, Khakoo R, Beezhold DH [2010b]. Measurements of airborne influenza virus in aerosol particles from human coughs. PLoS One 5(11):e15100.

Martinello RA, Jones L, Topal JE [2003]. Correlation between healthcare workers' knowledge of influenza vaccine and vaccine receipt. Infect Control Hosp Epidemiol 24(11):845–847.

Nafziger DA, Herwaldt LA [1994]. Attitudes of internal medicine residents regarding influenza vaccination. Infect Control Hosp Epidemiol 15(1):32–35.

Nichol KL, Treanor JJ [2006]. Vaccines for seasonal and pandemic influenza. J Infect Dis 194(Suppl2):S111–118.

Nichol KL, Hauge M [1997]. Influenza vaccination of healthcare workers. Infect Control Hosp Epidemiol 18(3):189–194.

Nichol KL, Lind A, Margolis KL, Murdoc M, McFadden R, Hauge M, Magnan S, Drake M [1995]. The effectiveness of vaccination against influenza in healthy, working adults. N Engl J Med 333(14):889–893.

Nicholson KG [1992]. Clinical features of influenza. Semin Respir Infect 7(1):26–37.

Norton SP, Scheifele DW, Bettinger JA, West RM [2008]. Influenza vaccination in paediatric nurses: cross-sectional study of coverage, refusal, and factors in receipt. Vaccine 26(23):2942–2948.

Nowalk MP, Lin CJ, Zimmerman RK [2008]. Self-reported influenza vaccination rates among health care workers in a large health system. Am J Infect Control 36(7)574–581.

REFERENCES
(CONTINUED)

ODJFS (Ohio Department of Job and Family Services) [2009]. Annual child care licensing report: state fiscal year 2009. Columbus, OH: Ohio Department of Job and Family Services, Office of Families and Children, Bureau of Child Care and Development. [http://jfs.ohio.gov/cdc/docs/2009%20Licensing%20Report.pdf]. Date accessed: October 2010.

ODJFS [2010]. Search for Available Child Care Facilities. [http://www.odjfs.state.oh.us/cdc/query.asp]. Date accessed: January, February, and March 2010.

Ohrt CK, McKinney WP [1992]. Achieving compliance with influenza immunization of medical house staff and students. A randomized control trial. J Am Med Assoc 267(10):1377–1380.

Plennevaux E, Sheldon E, Blatter M Reeves-Hoche MK, Denis M [2010]. Immune response after a single vaccination against 2009 influenza A H1N1 in USA: a preliminary report of two randomized controlled phase 2 trials. Lancet 375(2):41–48.

Slaunwhite JM, Smith SM, Fleming MT [2009]. Increasing vaccination rates among health care workers using unit "champions" as a motivator. Can J Infect Control 24(3):159–164.

Strangert K [1976]. Respiratory illness in preschool children with different forms of daycare. Pediatrics 57(2):192–196.

Thomas DR, Winsted B, Koontz C [1993]. Improving neglected influenza vaccination among healthcare workers in long-term care. J Am Geriatr Soc 41(9):928–930.

Thompson WW, Shay DK, Weintraub E, Brammer L, Cox NJ, Fukuda K [2004]. Influenza-associated hospitalizations in the United States. JAMA 292(11):1333–1340.

U.S. Census Bureau [2010]. State & County QuickFacts. Washington, DC: U.S. Census Bureau. [http://quickfacts.census.gov/qfd/states/39/39061.html]. Date accessed: October 2010.

U.S. Department of Health and Human Services [2000]. Increase the proportion of adults who are vaccinated annually against influenza and ever vaccinated against pneumococcal disease. Objective 14-29. Healthy people 2010 (conference ed., in 2 vols).

REFERENCES
(CONTINUED)

Washington, DC: U.S. Department of Health and Human Services. [http://www.healthypeople.gov/document/html/objectives/14-29.htm]. Date accessed: September 2010.

Vajo Z, Tamas F, Sinka L, Jankovics I [2010]. Safety and immunogenicity of a 2009 pandemic influenza A H1N1 vaccine when administered alone or simultaneously with the seasonal influenza vaccine for the 2009–10 influenza season: A multicentre, randomised controlled trial. Lancet 2010 *375*(9708):49–55.

Vellozzi C, Burwen DR, Dobardzic A, Ball R, Walton K, Haber P [2009]. Safety of trivalent inactivated influenza vaccines in adults: background for pandemic influenza vaccine safety monitoring. Vaccine *27*(15):2114–2120.

Wald ER, Dashefsky B, Byers C, Guerra N, Taylor F [1988]. Frequency and severity of infections in day care. Pediatrics *112*(4):540–546.

Wright PF, Webster RG [2001]. Orthomyxoviruses. In: Knipe DM, Howley PM, eds. Fields virology. 4th ed. Philadelphia, PA: Lippincott Williams & Wilkins, pp. 1534–1579.

Acknowledgments and Availability of Report

The Hazard Evaluations and Technical Assistance Branch (HETAB) of the National Institute for Occupational Safety and Health (NIOSH) conducts field investigations of possible health hazards in the workplace. These investigations are conducted under the authority of Section 20(a)(6) of the Occupational Safety and Health Act of 1970, 29 U.S.C. 669(a)(6) which authorizes the Secretary of Health and Human Services, following a written request from any employer or authorized representative of employees, to determine whether any substance normally found in the place of employment has potentially toxic effects in such concentrations as used or found. HETAB also provides, upon request, technical and consultative assistance to federal, state, and local agencies; labor; industry; and other groups or individuals to control occupational health hazards and to prevent related trauma and disease.

The findings and conclusions in this report are those of the authors and do not necessarily represent the views of NIOSH. Mention of any company or product does not constitute endorsement by NIOSH. In addition, citations to websites external to NIOSH do not constitute NIOSH endorsement of the sponsoring organizations or their programs or products. Furthermore, NIOSH is not responsible for the content of these websites. All Web addresses referenced in this document were accessible as of the publication date.

This report was prepared by Marie A. de Perio, Douglas M. Wiegand, and Stefanie M. Evans of HETAB, Division of Surveillance, Hazard Evaluations and Field Studies. Data management support was provided by Denise Giglio and Elizabeth Smith. Statistical support was provided by James Deddens. Editorial assistance was provided by Ellen Galloway. Desktop publishing was performed by Robin Smith.

Copies of this report have been sent to the county Department of Jobs and Family Services, the county Public Health, the state health department, management representatives at each participating child care center, and the Occupational Safety and Health Administration Regional Office. This report is not copyrighted and may be freely reproduced. The report may be viewed and printed at http://www.cdc.gov/niosh/hhe/. Copies may be purchased from the National Technical Information Service at 5825 Port Royal Road, Springfield, Virginia 22161.

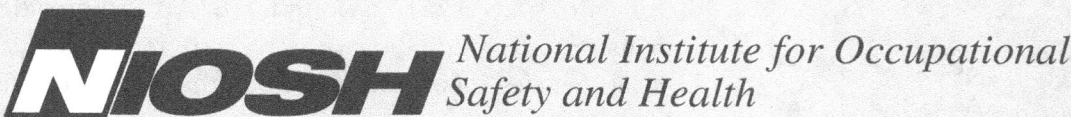

National Institute for Occupational Safety and Health

Delivering on the Nation's promise: Safety and health at work for all people through research and prevention.

To receive NIOSH documents or information about occupational safety and health topics, contact NIOSH at:

1-800-CDC-INFO (1-800-232-4636)

TTY: 1-888-232-6348

E-mail: cdcinfo@cdc.gov

or visit the NIOSH web site at: **www.cdc.gov/niosh.**

For a monthly update on news at NIOSH, subscribe to NIOSH eNews by visiting **www.cdc.gov/niosh/eNews.**

SAFER • HEALTHIER • PEOPLE™

www.ingramcontent.com/pod-product-compliance
Lightning Source LLC
Chambersburg PA
CBHW080911290526
45795CB00007BA/2498